Sildenafil Viagra Pills for Men

The Ultimate Guide on the Use of Viagra to Cure Erectile Dysfunction, Premature Ejaculation, Boost Libido and Peak Performance

D1430728

Dr. Leilani Cayman

Copyright @2022

Table of Contents

Chapter One

Introduction

Viagra is one of the drugs used to treat impotence. You cannot maintain or form an erection if you have ED. A male must be at least 18 years old to use Viagra for this purpose.

Viagra's active ingredient is sildenafil citrate. It belongs to the class of drugs known as phosphodiesterase type 5 (PDE5) inhibitors. Viagra improves the onset and duration of erections by increasing blood flow to the penis (a class of pharmaceuticals is a group of medications having similar mechanisms of action). You must be eager to engage in sexual activity in order to use this drug.

Oral Viagra pills are available. It is usually recommended that you take it an hour or two before engaging in sexual activity, although it can be taken up to four hours before. Viagra comes in three strengths: 25, 50, and 100 mg.

Chapter Two

How Viagra Works

Viagra begins to work between 30 and 60 minutes after taking the tablet. Viagra, on the other hand, does not produce an erection. Ecstasy abuse, on the other hand, must be sexual in order to be effective.

Viagra might take up to 5 hours to leave your body. If you take Viagra while you're hot, you should be able to keep an erection for up to 4 hours.

Even if Viagra continues to act in your body for several hours after you take it, your erection should not remain this long. In truth, some people may get priapism after taking Viagra. When you have this condition, you will have a lengthy, occasionally unpleasant erection.

Treatment for priapism should begin as soon as possible. If the problem is not resolved, the tissues in your penis may degenerate, leading to lifelong erectile dysfunction.

If your erection lasts more than four hours, go to the nearest hospital or call 911.

Chapter Three

Dose of Viagra

Depending on a few crucial circumstances, your doctor may advise you to take Viagra at a different dose. Among them are the following:

- ➤ Age
- ➤ Whether you have liver or renal problems,
- ➤ There could be further health risks.
- ➤ You may use a variety of prescription medications.

A list of common dosages or recommendations is presented

below. However, follow your
doctor's dosage
recommendations.

Your doctor will establish the
appropriate dose for you.

Drug Types and Strengths

Oral Viagra pills are available.
The dosage ranges available are
25, 50, and 100 mg.

**Most Effective Dosage for
treating Erectile Dysfunction**

The recommended dose of
Viagra for erectile dysfunction is
50 mg. Take this drug 30
minutes to 4 hours before
sexual activity. However, the
majority of people must take
their prescriptions around an

hour before engaging in sexual activity. Limit the number of Viagra doses you take per day to one.

Your doctor may advise you to take Viagra at a different dosage based on a variety of circumstances, including your medical history. You should think about any hepatic or renal issues you have, any drugs you're taking, and any other relevant facts. If you suffer any of these side effects, your initial dose may be 25 mg instead of the recommended dose.

Speak with your doctor if you have any questions regarding

your personal Viagra dose. If Viagra isn't working for you, your doctor may opt to increase your dosage. Viagra has a maximum dose of 100 mg.

Chapter Four

Side Effects

Viagra can have minor to severe side effects. The following are some of the most prevalent side effects that may occur after using Viagra. There are additional negative consequences besides those described on this page.

The majority of these side effects should subside within a few days or weeks. If they persist or worsen, see a doctor or pharmacist.

The list of Viagra's moderate side effects is not exhaustive. If you have any other minor side effects, read the patient information for the drug or chat with your doctor or pharmacist.

For further information on the potential side effects of Viagra, see your doctor or pharmacist. They can advise you on how to solve any problems.

The Food and Medication Administration (FDA) monitors negative drug responses. If you have any negative side effects while using Viagra, you can use MedWatch to contact the FDA.

Minor Adverse Effects

The following are the most prevalent Viagra adverse effects:

- ➢ Headache
- ➢ Flushing
- ➢ Indigestion
- ➢ Minor and transient eye illnesses include vision blur, light sensitivity, and a blue tinge.
- ➢ Nose congestion
- ➢ Dizziness
- ➢ Backache
- ➢ Nausea
- ➢ Muscle aches
- ➢ Rash

The majority of these side effects should subside in a

matter of days or weeks. However, if they persist or intensify, you should see a doctor.

Significant Side Effects

Call the medical emergency hotline if you suspect you are experiencing potentially fatal symptoms.

The following are some examples of obvious adverse effects and symptoms:

> NAION (non-arteritic anterior ischemic optic neuropathy), a problem with the optic nerve, has

an effect on the eyes. Among the indicators are:

> One or both eyes' vision rapidly deteriorates.

> Sudden loss of eyesight in one or both eyes

> Hearing loss that was unexpected

Other warning signs and symptoms of this illness include:

> Hearing loss and ringing in the ears

> Dizziness

The less enticing but more detrimental consequences are discussed further below.

> Reaction to Allergy

- Priapism (often unpleasant, protracted erections) (often uncomfortable, lengthy erections) (often uncomfortable, prolonged erections) (a lengthy, sometimes painful erection)
- When combined with other medications, Viagra can lower blood pressure.
- Heart attacks, abnormal heartbeats, and strokes are common in patients with cardiac illness.

Understanding the Consequences

You might be wondering how frequently specific adverse effects of this drug occur. A few of the drugs are covered in greater depth below.

Allergic Reaction

Viagra, like other medications, may cause unpleasant side effects in some people. Fewer than 2% of people in clinical studies, including Viagra, had an allergic reaction. The number of people who took a placebo and developed allergic reactions is unknown (no active drug).

Minor allergic reactions may result in the following signs and symptoms:

> ➢ Itching,
> ➢ Dermatitis,
> ➢ Rinsing (warmth and rosiness of the skin) (warmth and rosiness of the skin) (Skin warmness and rosiness) (You become hot and your skin turns red.)

More severe allergy reactions can occur, despite their rarity. The following are some of the warning signs and symptoms of an allergic reaction:

- Lips, eyes, hands, feet, and other body parts are commonly affected by edema.
- The lips, tongue, and nose are expanding.
- Breathing difficulties

If you use Viagra and experience a serious allergic reaction, contact your doctor immediately. Call 911 immediately if you suspect you are in a medical emergency or if your symptoms are severe.

Priapism

The priapism side effect of Viagra is characterized by a

long, sometimes painful erection.

However, it is unknown how frequently men who use Viagra get priapism.

Treatment for priapism should begin as soon as possible. If the condition is not addressed, the tissues in your penis may be destroyed, resulting in erectile dysfunction for the rest of your life.

If your erection lasts longer than four hours, go to the nearest emergency hospital or dial 911.

Low Blood Pressure

Your blood pressure may temporarily drop after using

Viagra. This, however, is frequently irrelevant. According to a scientific study, less than 2% of persons who used Viagra subsequently reported having decreased blood pressure. The prevalence of low blood pressure in patients who took a placebo (no active medicine) is unknown (no active drug).

If you take any other medications or have any other cardiac concerns, a quick drop in blood pressure could be dangerous.

For example, if you use nitrate drugs for chest discomfort, you should not use Viagra. If you are taking the medication riociguat, you should avoid using Viagra (Adempas). Because Viagra has the power to substantially reduce blood pressure, it raises your chances of suffering a heart attack or stroke.

If you already have low blood pressure, taking Viagra may cause agitation, dizziness, or even fainting. When you combine Viagra with several prescriptions used to treat high blood pressure or an enlarged prostate, your risk of acquiring these disorders rises. If you get lightheadedness or dizziness after taking Viagra, lie down until the symptoms pass.

Ask your doctor if taking Viagra is safe for you if you have a heart condition or low blood pressure.

For further information about mixing Viagra with other drugs, see the "Viagra interactions" section below. More information on using Viagra if you have heart or blood pressure concerns can be found in the "Viagra precautions" section below.

Stroke, heart attack, and irregular heartbeat.

Strokes, heart attacks, and irregular heartbeats are extremely rare in Viagra patients. Those with a history of heart disease were more vulnerable to these problems. The study discovered that even those who did not have heart problems experienced the same symptoms. It is debatable whether Viagra was the source of the negative effects.

If you have chest pain while using Viagra, stop using it immediately. If you suspect you are experiencing a medical emergency or if your symptoms are severe, dial 911 immediately.

Before taking Viagra, consult your doctor if you have a heart condition. You can ask them if it is safe to give you this drug. More advice on how to use Viagra if you have heart problems can be found in the "Viagra precautions" section below.

Headaches

Headaches are a common Viagra adverse effect. Headaches, flushing, and vertigo may be caused by the body's enlarged blood vessels caused by Viagra use. The medicine affects blood vessels other than those in your penis.

During clinical trials, between 16 and 28% of Viagra users experienced headaches. However, 4-7% of those who received the placebo reported headaches (this percentage varied depending on the dosage and pattern of Viagra usage).

You will not experience headaches for long after taking Viagra. If you're in discomfort, try taking an acetaminophen or ibuprofen-based pain reliever. Inquire with your doctor or pharmacist about a medication that may be appropriate for you.

If you get a severe headache or one that won't go away, call your doctor immediately once. They can help you make the best selection for headache therapy.

Older Men's Symptoms

Males over the age of 65 had higher post-dose levels of Viagra in their blood than younger men. As your blood medication level rises, your chances of experiencing unpleasant side effects climb. Older men, on average, use Viagra less frequently than younger guys.

During Viagra clinical studies, both males 65 and older and

males younger than 65 reported negative side effects.

If you are concerned about using Viagra at this time in your life, consult your doctor.

Chapter Five

Managing Adverse Effects

The majority of Viagra's minor side effects are tolerable or go away on their own within a few hours.

Remember that rest and sleep can commonly alleviate headache, flushing, and vertigo symptoms. By abstaining from alcohol, you can avoid these detrimental outcomes. You can lessen your sensitivity to light and gain headache relief by turning off any nearby bright lights. Speak with your doctor or pharmacist if you require a safe pain reliever while taking Viagra.

If using Viagra alone causes indigestion, consider taking it with a small snack or lunch. Just keep in mind that if you do this, Viagra may not start working as rapidly. If you experience indigestion, consult your doctor or primary care provider. (This is especially true if taken with a high-fat meal.)

Never underestimate the possibility that sustained Viagra use will result in more unfavorable side effects. Some of the negative effects include headaches, flushes, indigestion, nasal congestion, and vision impairment. If you are concerned about these side effects, consult your doctor about decreasing your Viagra dosage.

Keep in mind that some unusual Viagra side effects require immediate medical intervention. Seek medical care right once if any of the following symptoms appear:

➢ An erection that lasts more than four hours.

➢ During sexual activity, you may have chest pain, lightheadedness, or nausea that lasts after the sexual encounter but before you begin to relax.

- An abrupt loss of vision in one or both eyes.
- A sudden or severe loss of hearing.

Chapter Six

Precautions

If you have any other allergies, tell your doctor or pharmacist before using sildenafil. The inactive components in this product may cause allergic reactions or other complications. For further information, speak with your pharmacist.

Give your doctor or pharmacist a detailed medical history, especially if you have had a heart attack or a life-threatening irregular heartbeat in the last six months, chest pain/angina, heart failure, kidney disease, liver disease, high or low blood pressure, dehydration, penis conditions such as angulation, fibrosis/scarring, Peyronie's disease, a history of painful or protracted erections (priapism), or any other medical condition (such as retinitis pigmentosa, sudden decreased vision, NAION).

This drug may cause dizziness or blurred vision. You may experience lightheadedness if you consume alcohol or smoke marijuana (cannabis). Only drive when you are confident in your ability to do so safely. Never perform any work that requires concentration and sharp vision, such as operating machinery or a vehicle. Drink in moderation only. Inform your doctor about your marijuana use (cannabis).

Before any surgery, inform your dentist or surgeon of the products you use (including prescription drugs, nonprescription drugs, and herbal products).

Only use sildenafil during pregnancy if absolutely necessary. High pulmonary blood pressure during pregnancy is a risk that can harm both the mother and the unborn child. As a result, you should continue taking this medication until your doctor tells you to stop. If you intend to become pregnant, are currently pregnant, or suspect that you might be, talk to your doctor about the benefits and risks of using sildenafil.

Breast milk does not absorb this medicine well. Consult your doctor before beginning to breastfeed.

Chapter Seven

Interactions

Drug interactions may reduce the effectiveness of your therapies or increase your risk of major side effects. This book does not contain an exhaustive list of possible medication interactions. All of your medications, including over-the-counter, prescription, and herbal supplements, should be disclosed to your doctor and pharmacist. Never start, stop, or modify the dosage of a medicine without first consulting your doctor.

The chemical riociguat may interact with this drug.

When used simultaneously, sildenafil and nitrates can drastically reduce blood pressure. A rapid drop in blood pressure can result in lightheadedness, dizziness, and fainting. On rare cases, a heart attack or stroke may occur. A rapid drop in blood pressure can result in lightheadedness, dizziness, and fainting. On rare cases, a heart attack or stroke may occur. Butyl nitrite, amyl nitrite, and amyl nitrate are only a handful of the drugs known as "poppers" that are used to treat angina or chest discomfort. Never take sildenafil with any of these medications, including alcohol (nitrates like nitroglycerin, isosorbide).

While taking an alpha blocker, such as doxazosin or tamsulosin, to treat high blood pressure or an enlarged prostate/BPH, your blood pressure may drop too low, causing dizziness or fainting. Your doctor may recommend starting sildenafil at a lower dose at initially to reduce the chance of developing low blood pressure.

Other medications that slow the rate at which sildenafil leaves your body may reduce its effectiveness. Macrolide antibiotics (Clarivox, erythromycin), mifepristone, rifampin, ritonavir, saquinavir, boceprevir, and telaprevir are among them.

This medication should not be combined with any other pulmonary hypertension or erectile dysfunction (ED) medications that include sildenafil (such as tadalafil, vardenafil).

Chapter Eight

Overdose

If someone has overdosed and is experiencing serious symptoms such as fainting or breathing difficulties, call the emergency hotlines. If not, contact a poison control center right once. In the United States, phone 1-800-222-1222 to reach your local poison control center. A local poison control center is a valuable resource for Canadians.

An overdose can produce severe disorientation, sluggish or painful erections, and nausea. Please do not give anyone else this medication.

Chapter Nine

Storage of Drugs

Keep away from light and moisture in a dry, dark place. Avoid using the restroom. Never give drugs to pets or children.

Only flush or spill drugs down the toilet if ordered to do so. When the product is finished or no longer required, make sure you properly dispose of it. Contact a nearby drugstore or a junk removal service.

The End

Made in the USA
Monee, IL
03 March 2023

29086332R00024